Battle Against Your Insomnia

Vivek Kamath

ISBN-13:978-152399941

ACKNOWLEDGEMENT

I am grateful to my mother Late Mrs. Vimala Kamath for giving me the birth because of which I am able to attain this great moment of writing a book on "Battle Against Your Insomnia". My Mother died of Diabetes and Cardiac Aliment way back in November 2006. Today I am able to cure Diabetes, Heart Ailment, Insomnia, blood pressure, Cholesterol and any respiratory diseases thru Reiki healing method and many other diseases without Medicines. It was unfortunate that I do not have my mother with me. I am sure her departed soul will now be able to rest in peace today by seeing the achievement of her beloved son. My mother's love and affection was a key for me to attain this position today and instrumental in shaping up my life and destiny. I am very thankful to my mother for giving me this great opportunity to serve the world.

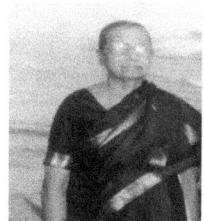

I would like to express my gratitude and heart-full of love to great Reiki Guru and Founder Dr Mikao Usui of Japan.

I would like to thank myself because of my inner strength with which I could able to convert the difficult situations or challenges faced in my life as a great opportunity for learning and always believed that life is a continuous education process. Furthermore, I strongly believed in my life that whatever happens in life it will happen for a good cause and these are based on our good and bad karma/action of past and current life.

Table of Contents

1 Introduction

Background about the Author

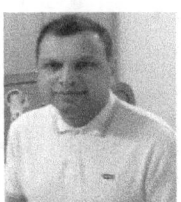

Author Vivek Kamath is an Indian Software Engineer by profession. Author has worked with the world's top International Banks across the globe for nearly 20 years to manage large scale Information Technology (IT) projects. Author is also a Reiki Healing Master Cum Practitioner and Practicing Reiki Healing, Mexican Healing, Crystal Healing, Melchizedek Method of healing from the last 5 years. Author has healed many diabetic patients, blood pressure patients (both high and low blood pressure), Heart Patients (removed the heart blocks), removed kidney stones , cured sinusitis, severe joint pains, constipation, migraines, headaches, insomnia, stomach related problems, diabetic gum problems, skin problems (dry skin, eczema) and chronic nasal allergies, nasal blockages without any medicines. Some of the above treatments have been completed within a week to maximum 1 month duration. Author has intention to help as much as diabetic patients to come out of the disease without any medicines. Author has an intention to build a healing center for diabetic patients across the globe.

For whom was this book prepared?

This book intended for people who are suffering from Insomnia problems. There are various Healing methods to heal insomnia permanently. Author has mentioned about the Reiki Healing in this book.

Author has intention to help as much as patients who are suffering from insomnia. Author has cured several patients who were suffering from chronic insomnia. In this book, author has given guideline how to heal your insomnia using Reiki healing method. If in case you are not able to heal by yourself, please feel free to contact author directly by email.

Author has used distant healing method (Patients can reside far away from the healer) of Reiki to heal some of the patients. Distant healing has been found to be very effective.

2 What is Insomnia?

Insomnia is difficulty falling asleep or staying asleep, even when a person has an opportunity to do so. If the people have insomnia they may below problems during the night

1. Difficult to fall sleep
2. Lie awake for a long periods at night
3. May wake up several times during the night
4. Some people may wake up early morning or midnight

and not able to get back to sleep
5. Not feeling refreshed when they wake up
6. They may feel tired and irritable during the day and have lack of concentration at work

What category of people who suffers from Insomnia?
1. Shift workers with frequent changes in shift
2. Elderly people
3. Patients who are taking aliphatic medicines for neurological disorders such as Parkinson's disease, schizophrenia, anxiety and depression
4. Frequent long distance travellers (those who change the time zone frequently)
5. Drug users, alcohol addicts and smokers
6. Pregnant women
7. Menopausal women
8. Patients who are taking aliphatic medicines for chronic diseases such as diabetes, high blood pressure, cholesterol, heart disease, kidney disease and thyroid problems etc.

Which is the key sleep inducing Hormone?

Melatonin is the principal hormone which induces sleep. This is a natural hormone produced by our body's pineal gland. The pineal gland is a pea-sized gland located just above the middle of the brain

Melatonin is called the "Dracula of hormones" as it only pops out in the dark. This hormone is essential for us to fall asleep. The pineal gland monitors changing light levels throughout the day and sensing the approach of nightfall, increases production of melatonin. Nighttime melatonin levels are 10 times higher than daytime levels. As we get older, not only does melatonin level drops down sharply, the timing of melatonin release also changes. Melatonin supplement will strengthen immune system function, improve sleep quality, stimulate release of growth hormone (GH)

How do we get sleep in the night?

During the day the pineal is inactive. When the sun goes down and darkness occurs, the pineal is "turned on" by the SCN (SCN is a small part in the brain expanded as "Supra Chiasmatic Nucleus") and begins to actively produce melatonin, which is released into the blood. Normally, this event occurs around 9 pm. SCN receives evening light from eyes and from our brain nerves. It is very important for people who suffer from insomnia to get light in the evening before the sunset.

Once melatonin levels in the blood rise sharply and we begin to feel less active and try to fall sleep. Melatonin levels in the blood stay elevated for about 10 hours - all through the night. Daytime levels of melatonin are hardly detectable.

3. What are the causes of Insomnia?

Examples of medical conditions that can cause insomnia are:

- Nasal/sinus allergies, Pollen allergies
- Un-health eating habits
- Gastrointestinal problems such as acidity or reflux
- Endocrine problems such as hyperthyroidism

- Arthritis
- Asthma and Chronic Respiratory diseases
- Neurological conditions such as Parkinson's disease and Schizophrenia
- Chronic pain
- Low back pain
- Allopathic Medicines taken for certain chronic diseases listed in below paragraph
- Jet lag
- People who switching working from day to night shift
-

Medications such as those taken for the common cold and nasal allergies, high blood pressure, diabetes, heart disease, thyroid disease, birth control, asthma, anxiety disorder and depression can also cause insomnia.

4. Symptoms of Insomnia

Below are some of the symptoms of Insomnia

1. Lack of concentration
2. Lowered mental alertness
3. Low IQ or Decreased problem-solving skills
4. Drowsiness
5. Inefficiency or decrease in efficiency
6. Nervousness
7. Irritability
8. Anger
9. Increased anxiety
10. Feeling depressed always
11. Fatigue, lowered physical performance
12. Frequent mood swings.

5. Global Fact Findings – Insomnia

1. According to a survey by the National Sleep Association, 22% of US people say they experience insomnia almost every night.

2. 27% of working women in the U.S. have insomnia, compared to 20% of working men.

3. About 30% of Americans complain of having insomnia.

4. About 1 in 4 U.S. Workers Has Insomnia

5. In USA, workplace Sleepiness Costs $63 Billion a Year in Lost Productivity

6. In United Kingdom, one out of 10 Britons can't fall asleep at night

7. An estimated one third of people in Europe suffer from sleep problems, especially insomnia. But only 20% get medical treatment.

8. In Australia, almost 1 in 5 people sleep less than 6 hours a night.

9. More than 20% of people with arthritis, asthma, back problems or diabetes reported symptoms of insomnia.

10. 23% of people who described their days as 'extremely stressful' reported insomnia.

6. Complications of Insomnia

1. Reduced performance at school and work

According to some research study, many people with insomnia are constantly tiered and unable to concentrate. This can lead to poor performance at work or school. The sleep-deprived often behave badly toward others. This factor and reduced performance, behavioral problems can damage professional and educational careers.

2. Risk of accidents

Chronic sleep deprivation slows response time and the ability to focus. This is how insomnia can cause both car accidents and accidents with commercial machinery at factory. People who have insomnia while driving have high risk of falling asleep and this can be just as dangerous as drinking and driving. These accidents often end in permanent disabilities or death,

3. Obesity

According to the Harvard Health Publications, living only on short bits of sleep can result in metabolic changes in the body. These changes may be linked to obesity.

4. Neurological disorders such as depression and anxiety

There are many psychological health disorders that can contribute to insomnia. Examples include post-traumatic stress disorder and bipolar disorder. There are also possibilities that chronic insomnia for a long time can bring on depression and anxiety.

7. Allopathic Medicines & it's side effects

In the table below, I have highlighted some of the Insomnia drugs with different trade name and their side effect.

Medicine Name/Drug Name	Side Effects
Doxylamine Eszopiclone Fluazepam Nitrazepam Zalepon Zopiclone	Melatonin side effects may include low body temperature, headache, nightmares and worsening of depression. It should be used with caution in individuals who have epilepsy, are taking warfarin (Coumadin), have autoimmune or endocrine disorders, or are pregnant or breastfeeding. Ramelteon side effects may include liver toxicity, dizziness, nausea, fatigue, headache and worsening insomnia.

8. Cure for Insomnia

There are several methods to cure Insomnia without medicines.

Below are the some of the healing techniques used across the world to cure insomnia problems. I am highlighting only Reiki Healing and Relevant Yoga's and Mudra's to heal the sleep problems.

   A. Reiki Healing

   B. Crystal Healing

   C. Pranic Healing

   D. Mexican Healing

   E. Holographic Healing

   F. Yoga and Mudra

Reiki Healing for Insomnia

A.   Reiki Healing

Reiki is a form of alternative medicine developed in 1922 by Japanese Buddhist Dr. Mikao Usui.

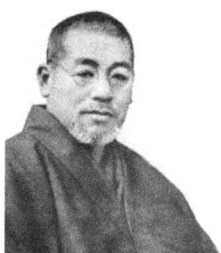

Mikao Usui 臼井甕男(1865–1926)

It uses a technique commonly called palm healing or hands-on-healing.The word Reiki is made of two Japanese words – Rei which means "God's Wisdom or the Higher Power" and Ki which means "life force energy". So Reiki is actually "spiritually guided life force energy or universal energy".

Any problem related to brain can be completely healed using Reiki Healing. Distant Healing (Patients need not be present in the physical location of the healer/Reiki Practitioner) method found to be very effective. Our mind governs the entire body and organs. In terms of Chakra healing, Reiki healer needs to heal the crown chakra of the patient. Also, healer needs to focus on healing the entire brain, glands and hormones. Healer needs to verify the patients report/patients inputs and check whether Insomnia is due to any existing chronic disease or whether existing disease's medication. If the disease is due to existing chronic disease healer needs to heal that disease first and make the patients to come out of medications of that disease. Healer also needs to heal the organs specific to existing disease.

With the Reiki, we can set the body clock and timer for removing the negative energies for the life time from the brain and penal gland. By doing this, we can permanently cure any chronic insomnia or any disease related to brain and crown chakra.

Yoga For Insomnia

Yoga is a Sanskrit word meaning "union" and is about getting the mind and the body to work together to find balance, harmony and ultimately better health .Yoga is Physical, mental and spiritual practice or discipline which originated in India. Yoga Gurus from India introduced yoga to the western countries.

In 1980's yoga became popular as a system of physical exercise across the western world. Yoga in Indian Traditions, however is more than physical exercise, it has a meditative and spiritual core.

Yoga can help to calm the mind, which is more important than you probably realize. One of the reason for the insomnia may be a constant source of worry and stress for varying different reasons. Yoga can help you to relax (both mentally and physically) and forget any worries through breathing and meditation.

Yoga moves can specifically help to cleanse the brain and rejuvenate the brain cells, heal the glands and hormones. With regular practice, yoga could help to keep your mind calm working at its best, and prevent any sleep or stress related issues. Please refer to appendix C for the list of yoga's are useful for Insomnia

9. Heal Your Insomnia in 3 Simple Steps

In Nut-shell Below are the Insomnia healing summary you may need to keep in mind.

Food Diet

1. Follow the Appendix A and B food to eat and not to eat for Insomnia

2. Always make a habit of drinking 3 Liters of water on daily basis. This will help to release the toxic or negative energies from our body.

3. Reduce Smoking and In-take of Alcohol. Smoking and alcohol blocks negative energies in your Ajna/eye brow chakra and crown chakra and elevates insomnia problems.

4. Nicotine in the cigars and caffeine in the coffee destroys sleep inducing melatonin hormones.

Exercise

1. Conduct those Yoga which helps to calm the mind healing (provided in book please refer to appendix)

2. Ensure you walk every day for 30 to 45 minutes.

3. Ensure your eyes get evening light (before the sun set) so that SCN (small part in your brain) passes the information to all other part of the body to shut their clock and turn off.

Life Style Changes

1. Practice Yoga or Meditation to reduce your stress, depression and anxiety levels

2. Practice some stress management techniques to reduce stress level

3. If you have time, practice 7 Chakra Meditation weekly once

4. Practice Insomnia Mudra for 15 minutes daily or thrice a week

5. Practice some deep breathing exercises helps to ease the blood flow in the brain and body circulatory system

6. Practice Reiki Healing on weekly basis helps you to balance all 7 Chakras which keeps you in good mental and physical health

7. Heal your Crown and Ajna/Eye Brow Chakra on regular basis to heal the brain. Ensure you cleanse the negativity from the mind on daily basis by healing Ajna/Eye brow and Crown Chakras. If you follow this on regular basis, you will not have any sleep problems This healing should take care of your any problem related to brain.

8. Follow the additional tips provided in appendix E

Appendix A Food to be taken manage Insomnia/Good Sleep

	Food	Description
1	Walnuts	Walnuts are a good source of tryptophan, a sleep-inducing amino acid that helps make serotonin and melatonin.
2	Almonds	Almonds are rich in magnesium, a mineral needed for good quality sleep.
3	Pistachio Nuts	High in Vitamin B6 helps to induce good sleep.
3	A slice of cheese or a glass of milk	Calcium helps the brain use the tryptophan found in dairy products to manufacture sleep-enhancing melatonin.
4	Lettuce	Lettuce contains lactucarium, which has sedative properties and affects the brain similarly to sleeping pills.
5	Fish (Tuna, Salmon, Sardines and Mackerel)	Fish mentioned here are high in vitamin B6, which our body needs to make melatonin and serotonin.
6	White Rice	White rice has a high glycemic index, so eating it will significantly reduce the time it takes you to fall asleep (Try Jasmine Rice For

		Faster Sleep)
7	Cherry Juice	Cherries, particularly tart cherries, naturally boost levels of melatonin.
8	Chick Peas	Chickpeas are also a good source of tryptophan can help to get good sleep.
9	Chamomile Team	Steeping a cup of chamomile tea will help you sleep. Chamomile tea is associated with an increase of glycine, a chemical that relaxes nerves and muscles and acts like a mild sedative.
10	Passion Fruit Tea	The Harman alkaloids chemicals found in high levels in the flower act on your nervous system to make you tired.
11	Honey	The natural sugar found in honey slightly raises insulin and allows tryptophan can help to get good sleep.
12	Kale, Spinach mustard green and other green vegetable	Green leafy vegetables like kale are loaded with calcium, which helps the brain use tryptophan to manufacture melatonin.
14	Grapefruit	Grapefruit is a great source of sleep-friendly B-Vitamins and dietary fibre. A grapefruit is a potent source of lycopene, a

		pigment that has been linked to healthier sleeping patterns.
15	Bananas	Bananas are a good source of potassium and magnesium, which both act as muscle relief and relaxants. Bananas contain Vitamin B6, an important micronutrient that aids in the body's production of serotonin, a trigger to the other sleep hormone melatonin.
16	Whole Grains	Whole meal Breads, oatmeal and cereal with whole grains are complex carbohydrates that help in increasing serotonin production.
17	Sweet Potatoes	Sweet potatoes contain B6, and a trigger for sleep inducing complex carbohydrates.
18	Food (Which are high in carbohydrates & high glycemic foods)	Carbohydrate rich food may help to get good sleep during the night. However, if you are suffering from high blood pressure, cholesterol, heart disease, kidney disease or diabetes it is not advisable to have high carb diet.

Appendix B Food to be avoided for Insomnia

Type of Food/Beverages

1   Deep Fried Foods

2   Micro wave Food & Fast Foods

3   Red Meat

4   Alcohol

5   Energy Drinks (sweetened fruit drinks, soda, and sports drinks)

6   Canned Food

7   Processed Food

8   Coffee, Tea – Stop taking 5 hours before the bed

9   Foods which are rich in protein need to be avoided 4 hours before the bed time

Appendix C Pranayama & Yoga for Insomnia

I have not documented how to perform these yoga steps in this book. I would advise readers to check with your professional yoga teacher and perform these yoga asana's/poses and pranayama's under their guidance.

Yoga for Insomnia

Please perform the below yoga or pose with the help of your yoga instructor. These yoga will be very useful to cure your insomnia. Also perform the breathing technique (pranayama) given below

1. Upavistha Konasana
2. Salabhasana
3. Viparita Karani
4. Supta Baddha Konasana
5. Jathara Parivartanasana
6. Savasana

Pranayama/Breathing Technique

Deep breathing techniques like bhastrika pranayama is very useful for insomnia.

Appendix D Mudra Insomnia

Please note the below mudra's for heart diseases.

Shakti Mudra

Shakti Mudra is good for inducing sleep. If we practice this regularly, it helps people suffering from chronic insomnia. To do Shakti mudra, join ring fingers and little fingers as indicated in the below diagram. The index and middle fingers will fold loosely over the thumb. The thumb will be bent inside the palm. Please see below snap boy performing Shkti Mudra.

Close your eyes and do Shakti mudra for 10-15 minutes. Slowly, visualize the physical and mental tension melting away.

Benefits: It cures Insomnia and also menstruation problems

in women

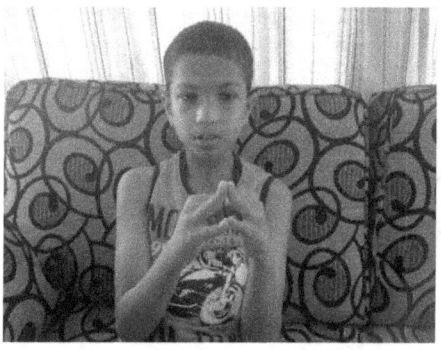

Appendix E Additional Tips for Good Sleep

- It is very important to set a regular times for going to bed and same with waking up in the morning
- Relaxing before your bed time a) Listen to good soothing music of your choice
- Male a habit of taking a warm bath before going to bed
- Using thick curtains o an eye mask and earplugs to stop you being woken up by neighbors light and noise
- Avoiding coffee, tea, alcohol, heavy meals before going to bed
- A light snack with a glass of milk and small banana or walnuts before bedtime may help to induce good sleep
- Avoid watching TV or working on computes just before going to bed
- Avoid sleeping during the day time
- Ensure you take a small walk before the sunset so that your eyes will get evening sun light this could help you to get a good sleep in the night
- Make your bedroom comfortable. Be sure that it is dark, quiet, clean and not too warm or too cold.
- Ensure you go out for a short evening walk to catch evening light (before the sunset)
- Keep your both the legs in the tub of lukewarm rock salt water for 20 minutes before going to bed.